PRAYERS & RITUALS AT A TIME
OF ILLNESS & DYING

PRAYERS & RITUALS

AT A TIME OF
ILLNESS & DYING

THE PRACTICES OF FIVE
WORLD RELIGIONS

PAT FOSARELLI

TEMPLETON FOUNDATION PRESS
WEST CONSHOHOCKEN, PENNSYLVANIA

Templeton Foundation Press
300 Conshohocken State Road, Suite 670
West Conshohocken, PA 19428
www.templetonpress.org

*Templeton Foundation Press helps intellectual leaders and others learn
about science research on aspects of realities, invisible and intangible. Spiritual realities include unlimited love, accelerating creativity, worship, and
the benefits of purpose in persons and in the cosmos.*

Designed and typeset by Gopa and Ted2, Inc.

Library of Congress Cataloging-in-Publication Data

Fosarelli, Patricia D.
Prayers and rituals at a time of illness and dying : the practices of five
world religions / Pat Fosarelli.
p. cm.
Includes bibliographical references and index.
ISBN-13: 978-1-59947-146-4 (alk. paper)
ISBN-10: 1-59947-146-9 (alk. paper)
1. Terminally ill—Prayers and devotions. I. Title.
BL625.9.S53F67 2008
203'.8—dc22
2008015314

Printed in the United States of America

08 09 10 11 12 13   10 9 8 7 6 5 4 3 2 1

CONTENTS

....

Introduction	vii
1. Buddhism	3
2. Christianity	17
3. Hinduism	43
4. Islam	55
5. Judaism	69
Concluding Thoughts	79
Notes	83
Bibliography	91

INTRODUCTION

....

IN MY ROLE as a teacher of theology students, chaplaincy students, seminarians, and lay visitors to the ill, I am often asked questions, most of which have answers readily available in books, articles, or on Web sites. Recently, a number of my students posed the same questions: What does one do when one is the first person on the scene of an urgent situation involving a person who is not of the student's faith tradition, and a cleric or lay minister of that tradition is unavailable? What should one do or not do? Over the years, I have told students that if they search hard enough, they would find answers to those questions, probably in some little handbook. All they needed to do was look.

In this case, I was wrong. Although there are (and have been) handbooks on what various faith traditions do in times of illness, they didn't necessarily include enough information to see why the practices flowed from the beliefs, and they didn't include prayers of the traditions that are important in times of illness or loss in terms of providing spiritual comfort. The books that have included such information are usually too large to carry around, which means that when one needed the prayers most, they weren't easily accessible.

This small handbook presents the spiritual beliefs, practices, and prayers of the five major world religions (Buddhism, Christianity, Hinduism, Islam, and Judaism) surrounding illness, dying, and death; the book's small size means that it can be carried in a pocket or purse for easy access. The purpose of the handbook is to acquaint those who care for the ill and dying—in hospitals, hospices, nursing homes, etc.—with each religion's basic tenets as to why illness and death occur and the practices that are sources of comfort to the ill/dying person and his/her family. Since religious practices flow from beliefs, it is helpful and sometimes imperative for one to be acquainted with the beliefs that undergird the practice in question.

I myself did research on each faith tradition through review of printed material and communication with practitioners of each tradition to determine what practices are usually done and what modifications must be made in a Western hospital setting. Whenever different branches of a religion vary in practice, these are noted. In addition, there are also sections for each religion as to what should not be done by one making a visit and any special prayers or practices for children.

In our modern pluralistic society, there are multiple religions practiced by the members of our population. Many individuals are married to those who do not share their faith tradition. Ideally, such couples adapt and adjust to each other's beliefs. Yet, even with adaptation, differences in prayer or practices might become a divisive issue at times of illness, dying, death, and loss, when what one individual needs is not what his or her partner needs in terms of spiritual support and comfort. When health or religious professionals encounter such couples at these difficult times, they might be concerned about the best way to proceed. It is important for those working with individuals at the particularly vulnerable times of illness, death, and loss to be aware of and sensitive to systems of beliefs that might seem foreign. Those who need to be particularly sensitive in this area would include those routinely making visits to the ill and dying or ministering to their families, such as chaplains, clergy, designated lay visitors, and staff persons at medical facilities.

At times of illness, especially terminal illness, religious practices should serve as a unifying force and not as a divisive one. When we are most vulnerable in terms of life's struggles and tragedies, our belief in God should be a help and not a hindrance. If that is true for us who minister, it is also true for those to whom we minister. As we understand the different beliefs and practices that the major world religions have in connection with illness or dying, we are better able to serve those who most need to be served. When we better understand which religious practices are essential and which are not essential, we go a long way toward meeting the needs of families and patients, for we can try to permit those that are essential and at least some that are not. Even when we cannot permit a certain practice because of regulations in Western hospital settings (e.g., burning incense when oxygen is in use), we can respectfully explain why such a practice cannot be done and look for practices that can.

Having respect for another's belief does not mean, of course, that one is not holding firmly to one's own beliefs or that one is trying to homogenize all belief systems so that they seem to be all the same. They are not all the same and never will be. Each religion has its own identity, and efforts to blur or minimize differences is dangerously naïve and erroneous. We cannot homogenize the essence of the various world religions without losing their distinctive marks, marks for which adherents have dedicated their lives or even for which they have died. That would be to trivialize that which is of utmost importance to millions of people.

Permitting an ill or dying person (or his/her family) to engage in spiritual rituals that have particular meaning to them does not imply that we are being unfaithful to our own religion. It simply means that we are secure enough in our own beliefs in God that we permit others to be secure in theirs. In the end, it means respecting others, a major tenet of every major religion. Mutual respect is important at all times, but especially so when one is vulnerable, such as times of illness, dying, or loss.

Many practices seem strange to us because they are not our own, but they are not strange to those for whom they bring comfort. For those individuals, it is *our* practices or rituals that seem strange. If we really cannot be open and present at such times to the practices and prayers of a tradition not our own, it is best to enlist someone who can, especially someone who shares the person's belief system. In a critical situation in which one individual holds a certain belief while the partner holds another, representatives of both traditions might be necessary. For example, a Christian is married to a Buddhist, who is terminally ill. Chanting before a picture of the Buddha, especially in the presence of a Buddhist priest, monk, or nun, might be important to both the patient and his spouse. Yet, the spouse might also need the presence of her minister for her spiritual care and comfort.

Being familiar with persons of various faith traditions is not just good for the persons in need. Trusted colleagues from different religious traditions can not only teach us about their religions, but they can also teach us something about ourselves and our own reactions to their beliefs. That is why it is vitally important to have relationships with persons from varying religious traditions, clergy or lay. Being in communication with those from faith traditions not our own also encourages ecumenical and interfaith dialogue and respect, activities that we desperately need in large measure in our often troubled world, a world that seems more often to be divided because of religion than united.

Prayers & Rituals at a Time of Illness & Dying

1. BUDDHISM

BUDDHISM was founded by Siddhartha Gautama, a prince of the fifth century BCE, who was protected from the harshness of life by his father, who kept him in the palace. Once the prince became an adult, he left the palace and encountered three people: an old person, an ill person, and a deceased person. The experience deeply affected him, and he became a "wandering seeker,"[1] searching for the truth that would free him from suffering. He tried many ascetic practices, but when he sat under a Bodhi tree (or tree of wisdom) and meditated, he finally saw reality as it was. He became the Buddha or the "enlightened" one. There are a number of branches of Buddhism, usually influenced by the culture in which they have emanated. Sacred texts for Buddhists include the Sutras (the discourses of the Buddha) and the Vinaya (the texts relating to the monastic way of life).[2] In terms of the latter, the Buddha felt that monks and nuns who followed his way were absolutely essential influences in the world.

BELIEFS

According to Christopher Partridge in *Introduction to World Religions*, Buddha taught that suffering (*dukkha*) results from ignorance of how things really are (*dharma*). Since change is always occurring, suffering results from trying to hold on to the present. Because life, as we know it, is changing and impermanent, clinging to it can only bring suffering, because everything must change and die. Buddhists believe that the self (*atman*) is a dynamic consciousness, moving from one body to another, according to karma (or the consequences of one's previous good and bad actions); that means, in Buddhism, there is no overarching "I" or self.[3] This movement from one physical body to another continues until one "lets go" and see things as they really are; if one "dies" when alive (as Buddha did), one discovers there is no reality to physical death.[4] Most Buddhists believe that one is reborn, not reincarnated, because there are ever changing mental and physical processes.[5] Death results in rebirths until greed, hatred, and delusion (which always lead to misery) are eradicated.[6] Once this occurs, one has attained nirvana, a state of perfect peace, where there is no desire and no awareness of a separate identity.[7]

According to Partridge, Buddha's Four Noble Truths are *dukkha,* which results from the emptiness of the existing order; craving, which is the origin of *dukkha*; the destruction of craving, which ends *dukkha*;[8] and the Eightfold Path (which Neville Kirkwood in *A Hospital Handbook on Multiculturalism and Religion* notes as right understanding, right thought, right speech, right action, right livelihood, right effort, right mindfulness, and right meditation).[9]

Compassion and wisdom lead to happiness, and so they are important aspects of Buddhist morality. Tenets of Buddhist morality include (1) never harming any living thing (compassion); (2) never taking what is not given; (3) never speaking falsely; (4) never engaging in sexual misconduct; and (5) never using anything that would cloud one's mind.[10] Buddhists try to achieve loving-kindness and tranquility through meditation, using their breaths or focusing on the present moment. All life is sacred and should be treated with utmost respect. Therefore, procedures such as abortion and euthanasia are against Buddhist beliefs.

ILLNESS AND DEATH: IDEAL PRACTICES

A health care provider of the same gender as the adult patient is usually preferred. When a Buddhist is ill, a visit from a Buddhist monk or nun should be arranged. The sick room should have a place for meditation before an image of Buddha.[11] Buddhists believe in organ donation as a supremely selfless gift to others.

Burmese Buddhists prepare for death by meditating on it during life; specifically, they practice anticipatory dying by meditating on (1) being about to be murdered, (2) the inevitable loss of achievements, (3) the weakness of all matter, and (4) the shortness of each moment.[12]

A dying person should lie on his or her right side, with legs gently extended.[13] It is important to die with a positive state of mind and to be at peace. A dying person's consciousness should not be clouded, and if administering pain medications would decrease consciousness, such medications might be refused. Those present with a dying person should provide hope and listen to him or her, perhaps whispering Buddhist mantras in the dying person's ear.[14] There should be no weeping or distractions. If strong emotions are present, Tibetan Buddhists believe that the deceased might remain attached to the present life, which would hinder his or her spiritual progress.[15] The dying person is encouraged to see all the positive things that he or she has done in life and to forgive self and others for any failings.[16]

In Tibetan Buddhism, the dying person should try, if possible, to visualize Buddha overhead, and his or her consciousness as a ball of fire rising up through the spine, leaving the head, and into Buddha. The *Tibetan Book of the Dead* should be read to the dying person so that he or she can move toward the luminosity that is the Clear Light.[17] In Zen Buddhism, the dying person (or those with him or her) says, "*Gate, Gate, Paragate, Parasamgate, Bodhi Svaha!*" which means, "Gone, Gone, Completely Gone, Totally Gone Through. Hail, Transcendent Wisdom!"[18]

Death practices vary by specific Buddhist tradition. Once the person has died, the body should be the rebirth. The casket is always open, and mourners should bow toward the body, but not touch it.[22] If a monk is not available, anyone can conduct the service as long as there is no reference to God (in whom Buddhists do not believe); in such a case, a eulogy is permitted, and passages from Buddhist scripture can be read.[23] Cremation is done within three to five days after death. Seven days after death (and at additional other times, according to tradition), monks chant from Buddhist scripture at the deceased's house to drive away ghosts, and to confer merit on the soul of the deceased to facilitate passing from the material to the spiritual world.[24] This "merit transfer" is facilitated by the deceased's family giving the monks food and gifts.[25] Since Tibetan Buddhists believe that there are forty-nine days between death and rebirth, prayers are particularly important in that time. According to their belief, the dead might not even realize that they are dead, and negative emotions because of fears, attachments, and grief might result in a less favorable rebirth.[26]

In most Buddhist traditions, ninety days after death, a memorial service is held, and another merit transference service is held on the one-year anniversary.[27]

Modifications on Ideal Buddhist Practices Based on Western Medical Routines

Because of any medical equipment to which the ill person is attached, he or she might not be able to lie on the right side, as is traditional. Also, incense would not be permitted in a hospital room setting.

Illness and Death in Children

Practices for children and adolescents do not differ markedly from those afforded adults.

Prayers

In the *Plum Village Chanting and Recitation Book*, compiled by the famous Zen Buddhist monk, Thich Nhat Hanh, there are many ceremonies for the ill, burial, cremation, and other events around the death of a person. For details about the ceremonies, the reader is directed to this book. There are no specific prayers for children listed.

A ceremony to support the ill would include (1) an opening ceremony (sitting meditation, incense offering, touching the earth); (2) a Sutra opening verse; (3) words about mindfulness of loved ones; (4) a passage about the Lotus of Wonderful Dharma; (5) introductory words (which may be amended as appropriate); (6) praise of the Bodhisattva of Compassion; (7) a wish for the day to be well; (8) words for protecting and transforming; (9) words for the three refuges (Buddha, Dharma, Sangha); (10) sharing the merit; and (11) words of gratitude (spoken by a relative of the ill person).[28] In both numbers 5 and 11, specific references to the ill person as child can be given.

Although the entire ceremony is a unit, the following words would be said during five parts of this ceremony:

Mindfulness of Beloved Ones

⋮ Brothers and Sisters, it is time to bring our beloved ones to mind; those to whom we wish to send the healing energy of love and compassion. Let us sit and enjoy our breathing for a few moments, allowing our beloved ones to be present with us now [ten breaths in silence].[29] ♥♥

Praising the Bodhisattva of Compassion

The Nectar of Compassion is seen on the willow branch held by the Bodhisattva. A single drop of this nectar is enough to bring life to the Ten Directions of the Cosmos. May all afflictions of this world disappear totally and may this place of practice be completely purified by the Bodhisattva's Nectar of Compassion.

Homage to the Bodhisattva Who Refreshes the Earth.

From deep understanding, the flower of great eloquence blooms: the Bodhisattva standing majestically on the waves of birth and death, free from all afflictions. Her compassion eliminates all sickness, even that thought of as incurable. Her light sweeps away all obstacles and dangers. The willow branch in her hand, once it is waved, reveals countless Buddha lands. Her lotus flower, when it blooms, becomes a multitude of practice centers. I bow to her. I see her true presence in the here and the now. I offer her the incense of my heart. May the Bodhisattva of Deep Listening touch us with her Great Compassion.

Homage to Bodhisattva Avalokiteshvara
[two bells].[30] ❧

Protecting and Transforming

: We, your disciples, who from beginning-
: less time have made ourselves unhappy out
of confusion and ignorance, being born and
dying with no direction, have now found confidence in the highest awakening.

However much we may have drifted on the
ocean of suffering, today we see clearly that
there is a beautiful path. We turn toward the
light of loving-kindness to direct us. We bow
deeply to the Awakened One and to our spiritual ancestors who light up the path before us,
guiding every step [bell].

The wrongdoings and sufferings that im-
prison us are brought about by craving, hatred,
ignorance, and pride. Today, we begin anew to
purify and free our hearts. With awakened wisdom, bright as the sun and the full moon, and
immeasurable compassion to help humankind,
we resolve to live beautifully. With all of our
heart, we go for refuge to the Three Precious

Jewels. With the boat of loving-kindness, we cross over the ocean of suffering. With the light of wisdom, we leave behind the forest of confusion. With determination, we learn, reflect, and practice. Right View is the ground of our actions in body, speech, and mind.

Right Mindfulness embraces us, walking, standing, lying down, and sitting, speaking, smiling, coming in, and going out. Whenever anger or anxiety enter our heart, we are determined to breathe mindfully and come back to ourselves. With every step, we will walk within the Pure Land. With every look, the Dharmakaya is revealed. We are careful and attentive as sense organs touch sense objects so all habit energies can be observed and easily transformed.

May our heart's garden of awakening bloom with hundreds of flowers. May we bring the feelings of peace and joy into every household. May we plant wholesome seeds on the ten thousand paths. May we never have the need to leave the Sangha body. May we never attempt to leave the sufferings of the world, always being present whenever beings need our help. May mountains and rivers be our witness in this moment as we bow our heads and request the Lord of Compassion to embrace us all [two bells].[31] ℰℐ

The Three Refuges

• I take refuge in the Buddha, the one who
• shows me the way in this life. I take refuge in the Dharma, the way of understanding and of love. I take refuge in the Sangha, the community that lives in harmony and awareness [bell].

Dwelling in the refuge of Buddha, I clearly see the path of light and beauty in the world. Dwelling in the refuge of Dharma, I learn to open many doors on the path to transformation. Dwelling in the land of Sangha, shining light that supports me, keeping my practice free of obstruction [bell].

Taking refuge in the Buddha in myself, I aspire to help all people recognize their own awakened nature, realizing the mind of love. Taking refuge in the Dharma in myself, I aspire to help all people fully master the ways of practice and walk together on the path of liberation. Taking refuge in the Sangha in myself, I aspire to help all people build fourfold communities, to embrace all beings and support their transformation [two bells].[32] ∽

Sharing the Merit

Reciting the sutras, practicing the way of awareness, gives rise to benefits without limit. We vow to share the fruits with all beings. We vow to offer tribute to parents, teachers, friends, and numerous beings who give guidance and support along the path [three bells].[33] ∽

A ceremony for burial or cremation would include (1) introductory words (which can be amended as appropriate); (2) consecration of the burial site or the crematorium, respectively; (3) contemplation on "no-coming, no-going" (i.e., that birth and death are illusions); (4) words at the burial or the cremation, respectively (which can be amended as appropriate); (5) recitation of Buddha's and Bodhisattva's names; (6) sharing the merit; and (7) hugging meditation and condolences. In both numbers 1 and 4, specific references to the ill person as child can be given.[34]

2. CHRISTIANITY

CHRISTIANITY grew out of Judaism. Jesus of Nazareth was believed by his followers to be the long-awaited Messiah. He taught the people about God's love and mercy and warned them to repent of their sinfulness. Because he emphasized love of neighbor above ritualistic observances of the Jewish Law, he came into conflict with the religious leaders of his day. One of his own disciples betrayed him to the religious officials who, in turn, handed him over to the ruling Romans on the charge that he made himself king of the Jews (and hence a threat to Caesar). He was executed by public crucifixion and was buried. Nevertheless, three days later, his followers reported that he was alive—not an apparition, since he ate in their presence. His once-fearful followers became emboldened proclaimers of his gospel (or "good news").

There are many different branches of Christianity. For the first thousand years, there was only one Christian Church, but a split between the Western (Roman) Church and the Eastern (Orthodox) Church destroyed that unity. Then, about five hundred years later, several Western Christians "reformed" the existing Roman Church. This was called the Protestant Reformation, and the multiplicity of Christian denominations continues to this day. For that reason, one cannot give information on the illness and dying rituals in every denomination, so general principles must suffice.

BELIEFS

Most Christian denominations believe in (1) God as Trinity—Father, Son, and Holy Spirit; (2) Jesus Christ as the Son of God; (3) the Holy Spirit's descent on the disciples at Pentecost, and the Spirit's role in the inspiration of the prophets and the church's inspiration today; (4) God as creator of all; (5) one baptism for the forgiveness of sin; (6) a judgment

ill to provide the sacraments, prayer, and emotional support. These sacraments include reconciliation (or confessing one's sins to a priest), communion (brought by a priest or lay person), and anointing of the sick by a priest. Prayer is important at the time of death in imitation of Christ who prayed both in the Garden of Gethsemane the night before he died and on the cross as he died.[1] In the Orthodox tradition, confession and communion are offered, although traditions differ on specific rituals to be performed. In mainstream Protestant churches, communion can be brought by an ordained or licensed lay person, and some Anglicans perform a final anointing of the dying.[2] In independent Christian churches, communion is offered, but there are no universal rituals at the time of death. Healing or anointing services are common, although some groups see illness as demonic possession that requires an exorcism.[3]

If an unbaptized person requests baptism, generally it is done by an official cleric of the denomination. If death seems imminent, anyone may baptize as long as water and a Trinitarian formula ("I baptize you in the name of the Father, Son, and Holy Spirit.") are used; this is true of Roman Catholics and mainline Protestant denominations. In the

Orthodox tradition, "any Christian priest or minister" may baptize in an emergency.[4] Independent Christian churches require a person to believe before baptism, which makes it difficult in cases of children. However, if parents consent, a dying child may be baptized. In churches that dedicate infants, this may be done by the appropriate cleric or chaplain.[5]

Neither Roman Catholics nor the Orthodox permit euthanasia, but extraordinary measures do not always need to be initiated or continued if death is imminent. The latter point is in agreement with other Christian denominations as well. Organ donations are acceptable to most, but not all, Christian denominations. Although most Christian denominations permit cremation, the Orthodox do not and will not offer a church funeral to anyone cremated.[6] All Christian denominations encourage family members to be present at the ill person's bedside and especially at his or her death.

Once death has occurred, the body is to be treated with great respect. In the Orthodox tradition, a body must be buried in a coffin in the ground, with a grave liner, and a cross to mark the grave.[7]

MODIFICATIONS ON IDEAL CHRISTIAN PRACTICES BASED ON WESTERN MEDICAL ROUTINES

None generally.

ILLNESS AND DEATH IN CHILDREN

As in most traditions, illness and death in childhood are great tragedies. Children are usually assumed to be far more innocent than adults, which makes their innocent suffering very difficult. Most Christians do not believe that young children are ill or dying because of their sins or the sins of their parents.

PRAYERS

In the Christian traditions, any of the Psalms can be used, especially Psalms 22, 23, 38, 41, 71 (for those of old age), and 88. Among these, Psalms 23, 41, and 71 convey hope, while Psalms 22, 38, and 88 describe feelings that the ill person may have.

In every Christian tradition, the Lord's Prayer, or the "Our Father" (the prayer that Christ taught his disciples), may be said:

Our Father, who art in heaven, hallowed by Thy name. Thy kingdom come; Thy will be done, on earth as it is in heaven. Give us this day our daily bread. And forgive us our trespasses [debts] as we forgive those who trespass against us [our debtors]. And lead us not into temptation but deliver us from evil. For Thine is the kingdom, and the power, and the glory, forever. Amen. ℰ℥

One major difference between Christianity and other world religions is that most of the major Christian denominations have prayers specifically for children, and some have rituals for them as well. It is beyond the scope of the present work to present all the prayers from every major Christian denomination, so an example or two must suffice.

Episcopalian

For a sick person:

O Father of mercies and God of all comfort, our only help in time of need: We humbly beseech thee to behold, visit, and relieve thy sick servant [NAME] for whom our prayers are desired. Look upon him/her with the eyes of thy mercy; comfort him/her with a sense of goodness; preserve him/her from the temptation of the enemy; and give him/her patience under his/her affliction. In thy good time, restore him/her to health, and enable him/her to lead the residue of his/her life in thy fear, and to thy glory; and grant that finally he/she may dwell with thee in life everlasting; through Jesus Christ our Lord. Amen. ✌

O God of heavenly powers, by the might of your command, you drive away from our bodies all sickness and all infirmity. Be present in your goodness with your servant [NAME], that his/her weakness may be banished and his/her strength restored; and that, his/her health being renewed, he/she may bless your holy Name; through Jesus Christ our Lord. Amen.[8] ✌

For an ill child:

Heavenly Father, watch with us over your child [NAME], and grant that he/she may be restored to that perfect health which it is yours alone to give; through Christ Jesus our Lord. Amen. ✌

Lord Jesus Christ, Good Shepherd of the
sheep, you gather the lambs in your arms
and carry them in your bosom: We commend
to your loving care this child [NAME]. Relieve
his/her pain; guard him/her from all danger;
restore to him/her your gifts of gladness and
strength, and raise him/her up to a life of service to you. Hear us, we pray, for your dear
[NAME]'s sake. Amen.[9] ⁊

For a deceased child:

O God, whose beloved Son took little children into his arms and blessed them: Give
us grace to entrust this child [NAME] to your
never-failing care and love, and bring us all to
your heavenly kingdom; through Jesus Christ
our Lord, who lives and reigns with you and
the Holy Spirit, one God, now and for ever.
Amen.[10] ⁊

For the parents:

Most merciful God, whose wisdom is
beyond our understanding; deal graciously
with [NAMES OF PARENTS] in their grief.
Surround them with your love, that they may
not be overwhelmed by their loss, but have

confidence in your goodness, and strength to meet the days to come; through Jesus Christ our Lord. Amen.[11] ✌

Lutheran

For a sick person:

⁝ O God, the strength of the weak and comfort of the sufferers: Mercifully hear our prayers and grant to your servants [NAMES] the help of your power; that their sickness may be turned into health and our sorrow into joy; through Jesus Christ. ✌

⁝ Blessed Lord, we ask your loving care and protection for those who are sick in body, mind, or spirit and who desire our prayers. Take from them all fears and help them put their trust in you, that they might feel your strong arms around them. Touch them with your renewing love, that they may know wholeness in you and glorify your name, through Jesus Christ, our Lord.[12] ✌

For an ill or deceased child:

God our Father, your beloved Son took children into his arms and blessed them. Give us grace, we pray, that we may entrust [NAME] to your never-ending care and love, and bring us all to your heavenly kingdom. Through Christ our Lord. Amen. ✌

Merciful God, comfort your servants whose hearts grieve and grant that they may so love and serve you in this life that, together with this your child, they may obtain the fullness of your promises in the world to come. Through Jesus Christ our Lord. Amen.[13] ✌

Methodist

Although extemporaneous prayers can be said at the bedside, the following are examples of more formal prayers from the Methodist tradition.

For an ill or dying adult or child:

Almighty God, we pray that [NAME] may be comforted, in his/her suffering, and made whole. When he/she is afraid, give him/her courage; when he/she feels weak, grant him/her your strength; when he/she is afflicted, afford him/her patience; when he/she is lost, offer him/her hope; when he/she is alone, move us to his/her side; [when death comes, open your arms to receive him/her]. In the name of Jesus, we pray. Amen.[14] ∾

For a dying person:

Gracious God, you are nearer than hands or feet, closer than breathing. Sustain with your presence our brother/sister [NAME]. Help him/her now to trust in your goodness and claim your promise of life everlasting. Cleanse him/her of all sin and remove all burdens. Grant him/her the sure joy of your salvation, through Jesus Christ our Lord. Amen.[15] ∾

At the moment of death:

Depart in peace, [NAME], in the name of God the Father who created you; in the name of Christ who redeemed you; in the name of the Holy Spirit who sanctifies you. May you rest in peace, and dwell forever with the Lord. Amen.[16] ∾

For a deceased child:

God our Father, your love gave us life, and your care never fails. Yours is the beauty of childhood, and yours the light that shines in the face of age. For all whom you have given to be dear to our hearts, we thank you, and especially for this child you have received to yourself. Into the arms of your love, we give his/her soul, remembering Jesus' words, "Let the children come unto me, for of such is the kingdom of heaven." To your love also we commend the sorrowing parents and family. Show compassion to them as a father to his children; comfort them as a mother comforts her little ones. As their love follows their hearts' treasure, help them to trust that love they once have known is never lost, that the child taken from their sight lives forever in your presence. . . . May things unseen and eternal grow more real for us, more full of meaning, that in our living and dying, you may be our peace. Amen.[17] ❧

Loving, heavenly Father, you have made us in your own image and likeness. We thank you for [NAME], for the richness of his/her personality, for the pleasure and love, laughter and tears that we shared together. We thank you that he/she is free from pain and suffering, and is at peace with you. God of all comfort, we give you thanks that Jesus took children in his arms and blessed them. Help us to know that Jesus has welcomed [NAME] into the kingdom of heaven. We make our prayers through Jesus Christ our Saviour. Amen.[18] ✏

For the parents:

God of infinite compassion, look in love and pity on those who mourn. Be their support and strength that they may trust in you and be delivered out of their distress; through Jesus Christ our Lord. Amen. ✏

Lord, listen to our prayers for this family who put their trust in you. In their sorrow, may they find hope in your infinite love; through Jesus Christ our Lord. Amen.[19] ✏

Orthodox

For an ill person:

⦂ O Lord our God, Who by a word alone did heal all diseases, Who did cure the kinswoman of Peter, You Who chastise with pity and heal according to Your goodness; Who are able to put aside every sickness and infirmity, do You Yourself, the same Lord, grant aid to Your servant [NAME] and cure him/her of every sickness of which he/she is grieved; and send down upon him/her Your great mercy, and if it be Your will, give to him/her health and a complete recovery; for You are the Physician of our souls and bodies, and to You do we send up glory: to the Father, Son, and Holy Spirit. Both now and forever, and to the ages of ages. Amen.[20] ⁌

For a terminally ill person:

⦂ Lord Jesus Christ, Who suffered and died for our sins that we might live, if during our life we have sinned in word, deed, or thought, forgive us in Your goodness and love. All our hope we put in You; protect Your servant [NAME] from all evil. We submit to Your will and into Your hands we commend our souls and bodies. For a Christian end to our lives, peaceful, without shame and suffering, and for a good account before the awesome judgment seat of Christ, we pray to You, O Lord. Bless us, be merciful to us and grant us life eternal. Amen.[21] ✌

For an ill child:

⁞ Heavenly Father, physician of our souls and ⁞ bodies, Who have sent Your only-begotten Son and our Lord Jesus Christ to heal every sickness and infirmity, visit and heal also Your servant [NAME] from all physical and spiritual ailments through the grace of Your Christ. Grant him/her patience in this sickness, strength of body and spirit, and recovery of health. Lord, You have taught us through Your word to pray for each other that we may be healed. I pray, heal Your servant [NAME] and grant to him/her the gift of complete health. For You are the source of healing and to You, I give glory, Father, Son, and Holy Spirit. Amen.[22] ✌

For a terminally ill child:

O Almighty God and Father of our Lord Jesus Christ, we pray to You for Your servant [NAME], whose sickness is bringing him/her to the end of his/her earthly life. You are the God whose only-begotten Son taught us that not even the smallest sparrow can fall without Your knowledge, and that You hold all creation in Your merciful arms. Look upon Your servant [NAME] and allow this illness to be the death only of those things which are the result of evil and sin. Let his/her thoughts be quieted with the peace and confidence of his/her final deliverance into the fullness of Your love. Keep his/her soul and body pure, and sanctify them during the time he/she remains among us, that on the last day he/she may be raised up with all Your saints to live with You in never-ending glory. For to You belong praise and worship, to the Father, Son, and Holy Spirit, now and ever, and unto ages of ages. Amen.[23] ✌

For a deceased child:

O Lord, Who watches over children in the present life and in the world to come because of their simplicity and innocence of mind, abundantly satisfying them with a place in Abraham's bosom, bringing them to live in radiantly shining places where the spirits of the righteous dwell: receive in peace the soul of Your little servant [NAME], for You Yourself have said, "Let the little children come to Me, for such is the Kingdom of Heaven." Amen.[24] ✑

For a deceased child by his/her parents:

⁝ Master, Lord my gracious and merciful God, ⁝ who long ago heard the grieving voice of Your servant Jacob, as he wept for Joseph, saying: I shall go, mourning, into the grave next to my son. You Yourself, O compassionate Lord, comforted David, the king and prophet, as he said in his grief: Absalom! My son, Absalom! It would have been better for me to have died in your place. O my son, Absalom! Your divine Son and our Savior, in His mercy for the grief which a parent suffers, raised Jairus' daughter and the son of the widow of Nain; and in this same compassion and loving-kindness, He healed the daughter of the Canaanite woman. O gracious and merciful Master and Lord, look down from heaven and behold the grief in my heart, the heart of a parent, as it sees its hope for life snatched away: the good and righteous life of my child through whom I had longed to praise the power, wisdom, and goodness of Your holy name. But as I stand before the impenetrable mysteries which You alone understand, my mind turns to the fervent prayer which Your Son, our Lord Jesus Christ, offered before the holy Passion in the garden of Gethsemane, saying: if it is Your will, take this cup from me! Like Him, I also bow my head before You today and cry out: Lord, let Your will be done! Like the righteous Job hearing of the death of his children long ago, I also cry out in humility and confess: The Lord gives, the Lord takes away; blessed be the name of the Lord. Though I am torn by grief, yet my faith in You and Your ineffable mysteries remains unshaken as I now beseech Your mercy and compassion, Lord. Grant forgiveness, Lord, to his/her soul for whatever sins he/she may have committed in word, deed, or thought; and bring him/her to that place of eternal blessedness, together with Your holy angels. At the time which You so choose, grant that I too may join him/her, so that together we may sing of Your immeasurable glory. For You are the God of mercy and compassion, and the Lover of mankind, and we offer glory, thanksgiving, and worship to You: the Father, the Son, and the Holy Spirit, now and ever and unto ages of ages. Amen.[25] ❧

At any time, the use of the Trisagion Prayers may be used:

⁞ Glory to Thee, our God, Glory to Thee.
⁞ O heavenly King, Comforter, the Spirit of Truth, Who art everywhere present and fillest all things, the Treasury of good things and Giver of life: Come and abide in us, and cleanse us from every stain, and save our souls, O Good One. Holy God, Holy Mighty, Holy Immortal, have mercy on us. Holy God, Holy Mighty, Holy Immortal, have mercy on us. Holy God, Holy Mighty, Holy Immortal, have mercy on us. ❧

⁞ Glory to the Father, and to the Son, and to the Holy Spirit, both now and ever, and unto the ages of ages. Amen. All Holy Trinity, have mercy on us. Lord, cleanse us from our sins. Master, pardon our iniquities. Holy God, visit and heal our infirmities for Thy name's sake. Lord, have mercy. Lord, have mercy. Lord, have mercy. Glory to the Father, and to the Son, and to the Holy Spirit, both now and ever, and unto the ages of ages. Our Father, who art in heaven, hallowed be Thy name. Thy Kingdom come; Thy will be done, on earth as it is in heaven. Give us this day our daily bread, and forgive us our trespasses as we forgive those who trespass against us. And lead us not into temptation, but deliver us from the evil one. For Thine is the Kingdom, and the power, and the glory, of the Father, and of the Son, and of the Holy Spirit, now and ever and unto the ages. Amen.[26] ∾

Presbyterian

For an ill person:

Lord of all health, you are the source of our life and our fulfillment in death. Be for [NAME] now comfort in the midst of pain, strength to transform weakness, and light to brighten darkness, through Christ our Lord. Amen.[27] ∾

O God, the strength of the weak and the comfort of sufferers, mercifully hear our prayers and grant to your servant [NAME], the help of your power, that his/her sickness may be turned into health and our sorrow into joy; through Jesus Christ. Amen.[28] ☙

For an ill child:

Jesus, friend of little children, bless [NAME] with your healing love and make [him or her] well. Amen.[29] ☙

For an ill child's parents:

Merciful God, enfold [NAME] in the arms of your love. Comfort [NAMES OF THE PARENTS] in their anxiety. Deliver them from despair, and give them patience to endure and guide them to choose wisely for [NAME] in the name of him who welcomed little children, Jesus Christ our Lord. Amen.[30] ☙

For a deceased child:

Almighty God, by rising from the grave, Jesus Christ conquered death and leads us to eternal life. Watch over [NAME]. Give him/her a vision of that home within your love where pain is gone and death shall be no more; through Jesus Christ, the lord of life. Amen.[31] ✑

Roman Catholic

For an ill person:

⁝ Father, your Son accepted our sufferings to ⁝ teach us the virtue of patience in human illness. Hear the prayers we offer for our sick brother/sister. May all who suffer pain, illness, or disease realize that they have been chosen to be saints and know that they are joined to Christ in his suffering for the salvation of the world. We ask this through Christ our Lord. Amen. ✑

⁝ All-powerful and ever-living God, the lasting ⁝ health of all who believe in you, hear us as we ask your loving help for the sick [especially NAME]; restore their health that they may again offer joyful thanks in your Church. Grant this through Christ our Lord. Amen.[32] ✑

For an ill child:

A service that includes a greeting; a reading from Mark 10:13–16 (Jesus and the children); a response to the reading (e.g., "Jesus come to me"); the Lord's Prayer; a concluding prayer ("God of love, ever caring, ever strong, stand by us in our time of need. Watch over your child [NAME] who is sick; look after him/her in every danger, and grant him/her your healing and peace. We ask this in the name of Jesus the Lord. Amen."); and a final blessing ("All praise and glory is yours, heavenly God, for you have called us to serve you in love. Have mercy on us and listen to our prayer as we ask you to help [NAME]. Bless your beloved child, and restore him to health in the name of Jesus the Lord. Amen.").[33]

For a deceased child:

⋮ To you, O Lord, we humbly entrust this child, so precious in your sight. Take him/her into your arms and welcome him/her into paradise, where there will be no weeping nor pain, but the fullness of peace and joy with your Son and the Holy Spirit forever and ever. Amen.[34] ❧

For the parents:

⋮ God of all consolation, searcher of mind and heart, the faith of these parents [NAMES] is known to you. Comfort them with the knowledge that the child for whom they grieve is entrusted now to your loving care. Amen.[35] ✌

3. HINDUISM

HINDUISM is unique in that it has no founder and no creedal statements. Yet, it is a four thousand-year-old polytheistic religion that has sacred scriptures. These scriptures are known as Vedas.

FOUR IMPORTANT PRINCIPLES

1. All beings are reincarnated over and over again (*samsara*). 2. The results of deeds done are visited on future lives (karma). 3. These endless rebirths are characterized by suffering (*dukkha*). 4. Liberation (*moksha*) from this suffering can only be achieved through spiritual knowledge.[1]

With regard to principle 1, there is no beginning and no end in time; it is cyclical. There is an endless cycle of life to death to life to death, and so forth. With regard to principle 2, the good (bad) deeds in one life have good (bad) effects in the next; the only ways to overcome karma is by devotion to a deity, religious rituals, and meritorious actions.[2] Otherwise, one is forced to work out in one's present life that which happened in a previous one.[3] Thus, reincarnation is affected by one's karma (past to now to future). When one lives an exemplary life, one is absorbed into Brahman, the ground of all Being.[4]

Death, then, entails rebirth according to karma over and over, until one finally achieves union with Brahman or one achieves a perfectly blissful state with liberation in paradise. Hence, the cycle of reincarnations is not meant to be permanent; it is only temporary.

Beliefs

The ultimate god in the Hindu tradition is Brahman, the ground of all Being. God is also understood in a three-fold way: Brahma (the creator), Vishnu (the sustainer), and Shiva (the destroyer and regenerator). Vishnu and Shiva are universally worshiped. Vishnu has appeared in the person of the avatars Krishna and Rama. There are also a multitude of lesser gods and goddesses who oversee various aspects of daily life.[5]

Hindus believe that God is within and also transcends every created being. "The essence of each soul is divine, and the purpose of life is to become aware of that divine essence."[6] One does this through meditation and grace. "One who knows Self puts an end to death."[7] This realization, known as *moksha,* liberates one from karma and *samsara.* In this way, *moksha* is salvation.

Even though the body dies, the self (*atman*) does not; even though physical bodies change, the True Self (*atman*) does not. The True Self is birthless and deathless; it cannot be destroyed. Those who die unaware of Self are reborn or return to lower evolutionary states because of karma. Those who die aware of Self are released from *samsara*, and immortality is finally theirs.[8] "When a person awakens and sees with a spiritual eye, reincarnation is no longer a necessity. . . . [One] wakes up from *avidya* (the ignorance of not knowing who the knower is), wakes up from karma (the impersonal law of causation in which action produces reactions), wakes up from *maya* (the illusion of separated identity), and realizes (Atman) True Self."[9]

How does one achieve this? One must die to all fears about living and dying. This is done by being attached to nothing—not this life, not the next. One surrenders entirely to God (Krishna), offering everything one does as a sacrifice to him. "Krishna reveals that one may be liberated from rebirth by being wholly concentrated, by keeping mind and heart united, by deeply surrendering to Krishna, and by uttering the mantra as one dies."[10]

ILLNESS AND DEATH: IDEAL PRACTICES

Illness is a result of one's karma. A good Hindu knows this and is expected to accept illness, frequently with the help of a Hindu priest. Incense is frequently used around an ill person. Either the patient or those around him or her can read from the Hindu scripture to assist in the acceptance.[11] In general, the eldest male member makes the decisions about care, but the entire family cares for the person. The diagnosis of a terminal condition is given to the family and not to the patient directly, and a family member will decide how much information the ill person will receive.[12]

If the person is dying, a thread may be tied around the neck or waist of the person; a leaf from a sacred bush may be placed on his or her tongue; and he or she may want to lie on the floor so as to be closer to the earth. Some Hindus believe that it is best to die on ritually clean ground, rather than on a bed, because a soul released from a height (at the moment of death) would be disoriented. Because one's final thoughts determine the first moments of the afterlife experience, it is important to surround the person with that which is holy. If available, water from the Ganges River, the holiest of Hindu rivers, may be placed in the dying person's mouth by a relative, while other family members chant Vedic mantras that are soothing in both sound and content.[13]

When death comes, the family should be consulted as to how the body should be handled. Family members prepare the body with a ritual washing and anointing. Any hair is trimmed and clean clothes adorn the body, (which remains at the home until it is time for cremation). Some do not wash the body, while others enshroud it or place it in a white sheet. Non-Hindus who handle the body must use gloves to close the eyes or to straighten the limbs. Death rituals are done by the eldest son to pay the debt owed to his ancestors and to the deceased;[14] if there is no eldest son, the eldest daughter or mother does the rituals.[15]

The funeral is within twenty-four hours. Mourners should wear white and bring flowers; they are not to touch the body in any way. The body is carried to the funeral pyre. Hindu priests or senior family members conduct the funeral service chanting Vedic funeral mantras. A food offering is made to the deceased before cremation.[16] The eldest son ignites the funeral pyre (under the head and feet) after pouring sacred water on the body. Cremation is performed because "[a]s long as the physical body remains visible . . . the soul remains nearby for days or months. The corpse is burned so that the soul can begin its journey as soon as possible."[17] Once the body is singed, the son takes a stick and cracks the deceased's skull to release vital air and the soul (*atman*).[18] The cremation continues in the belief that the fire of cremation is the final source of healing.[19]

Family members are ritually impure after death for three to sixteen days, or even longer. Once home from the cremation, family members ritually bathe, recite prescribed mantras, and offer libations at the family altar ten days. They can visit no one, can have no contact with people outside their family, cannot wash clothes, and they can only eat once per day. Three days after the cremation, the oldest son returns to the site of the cremation and either buries or casts into a river any remaining bones.[20] The family's period of pollution is closed by the *suddhi* feast.[21] The ceremony occurs ten or thirty days (depending on the caste) after the death at his or her home; the purpose is to liberate the soul for its ascent to heaven by encouraging family reconciliation and celebration.[22] In all of these actions, the soul is supported in its "journey to the next world, whether from one body to the next, or from this life to Eternal Brahman."[23]

Modifications on Ideal Hindu Practices Based on Western Medical Routines

Incense cannot be used in a hospital room setting.

Illness and Death in Children

There are no specific rituals for children, although children younger than twelve years are always buried.

Prayers

Prayers and practices for seriously ill or dying Hindu children follow general practices. Visiting a seriously ill or dying person and his or her family provides comfort in time of distress, especially speaking about God's holy will. Chanting of God's name at the time of death not only provides comfort to the dying person and his or her family, but it also is believed in Hindu theology that doing so will merit the dying person *moksha,* or salvation. Depending on the deity in which the family has the greatest faith, his or her name would be the one chanted, although the name of Lord Shiva can always be chanted, especially at the final moments. An example of a chant would be "Hari Krishna" or "Hari, hari." For very young or for persons who are unconscious, family members can do the chanting of the presiding deity's name. Ideally, a Hindu priest is present, but anyone who has knowledge of the Hindu scriptures can lead the chanting, although some families may only want a true Hindu believer to do so.[24]

Reading particularly apropos verses of the *Bhagavad Gita* can also be comforting. The following verses, translated by Mascaro, are attributed to Lord Krishna (God), as he spoke gently to the warrior, Arjuna, who was sorrowful over having to kill in battle.[25] His words underscore the impermanence of death and the importance of devotion to God.

Verses

Impermanence of death:

(2:11–13) The wise grieve not for those who live; and they grieve not for those who die— for life and death shall pass away. Because we all have been for all time: I, thou, and kings of men. And we shall be for all time. . . . As the Spirit of our mortal body wanders on in childhood, youth, and old age, the Spirit wanders on to a new body. . . . ☙

(2:16–17) The unreal never is; the Real never is not. . . . Interwoven in his creation, the Spirit is beyond destruction. No one can bring to an end the Spirit which is everlasting. ☙

(2:20) He is never born, and he never dies. He is in eternity; he is for evermore. Never-born and eternal, beyond times gone or to come, he does not die when the body dies. ☙

⦂ (2:22) As a man leaves an old garment and puts on one that is new, the Spirit leaves his mortal body and then puts on one that is new. ☙

⦂ (2:24–28) Beyond the power of sword and fire, beyond the power of waters and winds, the Spirit is everlasting, omnipresent, never-changing, never-moving, ever One. Inevitable is he to mortal eyes, beyond thought and beyond change. Know that he is, and cease from sorrow. But if he were born again and again, and again and again, he were to die, even then, victorious man, cease thou from sorrow. For all things born in truth must die, and out of death in truth comes life. Face to face with what must be, cease thou from sorrow. Invisible before birth are all beings and after death invisible again. They are seen between two unseens. Why in this truth find sorrow? ☙

Importance of devotion to God:

⦂ (2:47) Set thy heart upon thy work, but never on its reward. Work not for a reward; but never cease to do thy work. Do thy work in the peace of Yoga and, free from selfish desires, be not moved in success or in failure. Yoga is evenness of mind—a peace that is ever the same. ℰᕲ

⋮ (2:71–72) For the man who forsakes all desires and abandons all pride of possession and of self reaches the goal of peace supreme. This is the Eternal in man, O Arajuna. Reaching him, all delusion is gone. Even in the last hour of his life upon earth, man can reach the Nirvana of Brahman—man can find peace in the peace of his God. ℰᕲ

⋮ (8:2) [Arajuna asks Krishna: And when the time to go comes, how do those whose soul is in harmony know thee?] ℰᕲ

⋮ (8:5) [Krishna responds:] And he who at the end of his time leaves his body thinking of me [alone], he in truth comes to my being; he in truth comes unto me. ℰᕲ

⋮ (8:7–8) Think of me therefore at all times; remember thou me. . . . And with mind and reason on me, thou shalt in truth come to me. For if a man thinks of the Spirit Supreme with a mind that wanders not, . . . he goes to that Spirit of Light. ✑

- (8:15–16) And when those great spirits are in me, the Abode of joy supreme, they never again return to this world of human suffering. For all worlds pass away, even the world of Brahma, the Creator; they pass away and return. But he who comes unto me goes no more from death to death. ✑

- (8:20–22) Beyond this creation, visible and invisible, there is an Invisible, higher, Eternal; and when all things pass away, this remains forever and ever. The Invisible is called the Everlasting and is the highest End supreme. Those who reach him never return. This is my supreme abode. This Spirit Supreme, Arajuna, is attained by an ever-living love. In him, all things have their life, and from him, all things have come. ✑

4. ISLAM

ISLAM means submission, and a Muslim is one who submits. The sacred scripture revealed and dictated to the prophet Muhammad is the Qur'an. In the early 600s, Muhammad came to believe that he was receiving messages from God (through the angel Gabriel) that he was to share with his countrymen. These messages form the basis of the Qur'an. Muhammad's messages were not always well received because they were often critical of the way people behaved. He and his followers were persecuted, and they fled from Mecca to Medina, which was more receptive to the messages that Muhammad had received. He continued to receive messages in Medina. "It was in Medina that the religion of Islam took shape."[1] Once Muhammad died, two factions developed as to who should be his successor; these factions, which still exist today, are known as the Sunni and the Shi'a (also known as the Shiites). Most of the world's Muslims are Sunnis (85 percent).[2] There is also a smaller sect of Islam called Sufi, which represents a more mystical tradition.

BELIEFS

Muslims believe that God (Allah) is one, the creator of all. He is sovereign and provides all things; a believer's life belongs to him. Allah wills all that happens in a person's life. Thus, religious Muslims do not complain about life since that would be a complaint against Allah. They also do not show fear, as that would demonstrate a lack of faith and a lack of submission to Allah.[3]

Muslims believe in angels, special messengers, and prophets, the last great prophet being Mohammad.[4]

The five pillars of Islam are (1) *shahada*: the confession of faith—"There is no God but Allah, and Mohammad is his prophet"; (2) *salat*: prayer (facing Mecca) five times per day; (3) *zakat*: almsgiving of at least 2.5 percent; (4) *sawm*: fasting during the month of Ramadan; and (5) *hajj*: pilgrimage to Mecca at least once in a lifetime.[5]

Muslims believe in a day of judgment (when deeds are weighed on a scale—see below); the pleasures of heaven and the torments of hell are detailed in the Qur'an. Even the creation story in the Qur'an notes that death is inevitable and that there will be a day of judgment at the end. There is a barrier between the living and the dead, and the deceased have no way to return to earth; instead, they must wait for the day of judgment. On that day, the dead will rise from their graves, and all will be judged by the number of good and bad deeds they did while alive; the righteous will go to the right, while the sinful will go to the left. Those who are the most spiritually advanced will be "nearest to God."[6] In the end, a soul either goes to heaven or to hell; in the Muslim tradition, both are described with earthly delights or torments, respectively.[7]

To prepare for the day of judgment, one must die to self daily in order to gain intimacy with Allah. Everything, even one's self-identity is "extinguished into Allah."[8] "Allah then becomes the lover, beloved, and the act of loving itself."[9] One concentrates on loving God everywhere and in everyone; "God's nearness possesses one's heart."[10] In this way, one draws closer to Allah in all activities.

Because Allah wills death for every living thing and determines the life span for each thing, Muslims must accept the reality of death.

ILLNESS AND DEATH: IDEAL PRACTICES

Although one must be cognizant of dietary rules, the ill do not need to observe the Ramadan fast. Ritual washing must be done before prayer, and so a basin at the bedside should be provided for those who are bed-bound. If the person is too ill for even a light washing at bedside, a dry cleansing may be done. An imam visits the ill person and recites portions of the Qur'an with him or her; if an imam is not present, a family member may do the same. Christian clergy might be acceptable if no imam is available, since "Jesus is the only healing prophet in the Qur'an."[11] Many Muslims do not name the ill person in the prayers, since they believe that would demonstrate criticism of Allah's will; since hardship and death are the will of Allah, one must accept them.

When a person is dying, he or she should be supine and face toward Mecca (west to southwest from the

U.S.); the head should be elevated.[12] Anyone who is unclean or menstruating must leave the room. The Muslim call to prayer (*kalima*) and *Sura* 36 from the Qur'an are recited.[13] Allah is praised for his mercy and forgiveness, with the hope that the dying will receive them as well. The goal is acceptance of "perceived punishment" for what one has done or failed to do.[14] Thus, the dying person repents of all earthly sins. The words of the dying Muhammad are inspiring: "Suffering is an expiation for sin. If a believer suffer but the scratch of a thorn, the Lord raiseth his rank thereby and wipeth away from him a sin."[15]

Because of their belief in the resurrection of the body on the last day, bodies must be buried intact; Muslims do not permit cremation, autopsy, or organ donation.[16] Euthanasia is also not permitted because that would violate God's will.

Once the person has died, only Muslims of the same gender as the deceased can handle the body. If Muslims are not available, non-Muslims can handle the body, but only wearing gloves.[17] The practice of Muslims when a person dies is to close the deceased's eyes and say: "Oh God, forgive (NAME) and elevate his/her station among those who are guided. Send him/her along the path of those who came before and forgive him/her, oh Lord of the Worlds. Enlarge for him/her his/her grave and shed light upon him/ her in it."[18] Preparation of the body includes closing the eyes and mouth; taping the lower jaw to the head; straightening the body; not cutting nails or washing hair; binding the feet together; unclothing the body; and covering the body with a sheet. The family ritually washes, perfumes, and wraps the body in white cotton, while they and the imam pray. For the washing, cool, pure water, sometimes perfumed, is used. The head of a man is wrapped in a turban; the head of a woman is covered with a veil. In the presence of the corpse, there are prescribed prayers and gestures.[19]

After death, Muslims try to have the body buried as soon as possible, although sometimes that is impossible if an autopsy must be done. Muslims abhor any desecration of the body, so most Muslims would not agree to an autopsy.

A Muslim funeral lasts between thirty to sixty minutes and occurs two to three days after death. The site is at a funeral home or the home of the deceased, and the casket (always wooden) is never open. The officiant is an imam who reads from the Qur'an. Mourners wear dark colors as a sign of respect, and non-Muslims should not wear signs of their own faith tradition. Male mourners are separated from female mourners.[20] At the gravesite, the body is removed from the coffin and placed in the ground on its right side, facing Mecca, with support of the head and feet by earth or a brick. Mourners cover the body with flowers and three handfuls of dirt and pour blessed rose water over it. Although some Muslim communities do not mark the grave or permit, at most, an unadorned piece of stone or wood to mark the grave, grave markings are permitted by other Muslim communities as long as the markings are religious in nature.[21]

Grieving is done for three days. During this time, neighbors prepare food for the family. Emotional displays are discouraged. In some cultures, women have their own rituals during this time, but they are to be separate from those of the men.[22]

MODIFICATIONS ON IDEAL MUSLIM PRACTICES BASED ON WESTERN MEDICAL ROUTINES

It is important to keep the ill, dying, or deceased person decently covered to the greatest extent that such is possible.

Illness and Death in Children

In general, children are not treated differently than are adults in Islam; that is, there are no specific prayers or practices for children of any age.

Prayers

In his book, *Pastoral Care to Muslims,* Neville Kirkwood included several bedside prayers that had been contributed by the Islamic Council of New South Wales:

⋮ Merciful and Compassionate God, we bow ⋮ before you, in full submission. The weakness in body, mind, and spirit is filling [NAME] with dread. You have planned our days before we were born. You are the only God. Beside you, there is no other God. In your mercy, look upon [NAME] in his/her present condition. There is pain and other anxieties. . . . We bring [NAME] before you that you might exercise your great compassion on him/her. Ease the pain. Give him/her strength for each day's need. We ask this so that his/her mind will not be filled with problems of his/her body but will be concentrated upon you. May his/her thoughts be focused upon you as one who is in Islam. Keep him/her obedient to your will at all times so that on the Day, [NAME] will walk in the Garden. In the name of God—Bishmi'llah. ✂

All Wise, All-Knowing, Eternal God, You understand and know all that [NAME] is experiencing in these days of illness. His/her mind is so troubled that he/she may have displeased you. Look favorably upon him/her in this hour of illness and pain. We pray that you will relieve [NAME] of pain and stress. Fill [NAME] with the calmness that your peace can give to a person's spirit. All-knowing God, we beseech you to forgive and bless him/her as he/she lies here, committing his/her life into your control. Forgive, restore your peace, and grant [NAME] a safe passage across the bridge on the Day of Resurrection. In the name of God and according to your will—Insha'llah. ✂

You are the All-Powerful, Benevolent God. We come before you not with confidence in ourselves but with full trust in you. You are the All-Wise One who created [NAME], who is before us in pain of body, distress of mind, and fearful in spirit. His/her illness is taking its toll upon him/her. We ask, Oh! Holy One, that you will be pleased to give him/her patience to endure the pain in thankfulness to you. May strength to cope with each day's burdens be granted him/her. We ask this not for ourselves but that his/her faith in you and submission to your will may not falter. Grant that faith will be sufficient unto the day when you summon all before the Judgment. On that Day, may he/she be granted entry to Paradise. Insha'llah—in the will of God.[23] ☙

When a patient is dying, the following may be said:

⁞ There is no God but Allah, the Forebearing, the Generous. There is no God but Allah, the High, the Grand. Praise be to Allah, the Lord of the Seven Heavens and the Seven Earths and what is in them, between them, and beneath them. And the Lord of the great Throne, and praise belongs to God, the Lord of the Universe.[24] ☙

When death is imminent, the dying person (facing Mecca, if possible) says:

:: O Allah, forgive me, have mercy on me and
:: unite me with the Most High Companion.
. . . None is worthy of praise beside Allah.
Surely death has many hardships and difficulties. . . . O Allah, help me in overcoming the
throes and difficulties of death.[25] ✄

Once death has occurred, those in attendance
pray:

:: O Allah, forgive [NAME]; and raise him/
:: her status [in Jannah—the Garden] among
the rightly guided people; and be his/her representative among his/her people who he/she
has left behind and forgive us and him/her. O
Sustainer of the worlds. And (O Allah) make
his/her grave vast and accommodating and fill
it with light (*noor*).[26] ✄

As mentioned previously, children are not treated
differently than adults in Islam; that is, there are no
specific prayers or practices for them. The prayers,
as with any other prayer, are reported to be said by

Mohammad when he visited the sick. One prayer is this: "Oh, God, Lord of mankind, take away the suffering, bring about the cure. You are the Curer, there is no cure except your cure, the cure that leaves no traces of illness."[27]

Because Muslims do not believe that children acquire sin until they reach the age when they can discern between right and wrong (i.e., puberty), some of the prayers above that mention displeasing God might not be apropos. Prayers for children would ask that their pain, suffering, and anxiety would be relieved and they would enter the Garden, which Muslims believe is the inevitable fate of children who die before the age of puberty.[28]

If a child is old enough, he or she should be gently reminded to place his or her right hand over the site of pain or illness, saying the prayer below. If the child is very young or poorly conscious, the one saying the following prayer can do this. "In the name of God" is said three times and then "I seek refuge in the Might and Power of God from the evil of that which I am [you are] experiencing and that which I [you] fear" is said seven times. Or, "I ask God, the Mighty, Lord of the Mighty Throne, to cure you" can be said seven times by the one praying. Alternatively, one can say,

"In the name of God, the Most Compassionate, the Most Merciful, I seek refuge in God—the One, the Only, the One who does not beget, nor was He begotten, nor is there anyone like Him—from the evil of that which you are experiencing."[29]

5. JUDAISM

JUDAISM began with the call of Abram, a nomad, by God, who promised that he would make him a great nation. Abram left his country and went to the land promised by God. Because he was childless, his wife permitted him to have sexual relations with her servant, Hagar, who bore a son (Ishmael). Later, when Sarah bore a son, named Isaac, Hagar and Ishmael were cast away into the dessert. (As an aside, Ishmael is felt to be the ancestor of the Muslim people.) Isaac had two sons, Esau and Jacob. Jacob had an encounter with God in the dessert, and his name was changed to Israel. Israel had twelve sons, who are the ancestors of the twelve tribes of Israel. These tribes migrated into Egypt, but after a time, they were persecuted there. Moses, one of Israel's great prophets, was chosen by God to lead the Israelites out of Egypt to the Promised Land (Canaan). Thus began the saga of the Jewish people.

There are five branches of Judaism: Hasidism (ultra-conservative); Orthodox (very conservative, true to the Torah); Conservative (conservative and true to tradition with some adjustments); Reconstruction-ist (belief that Judaism is ever evolving); and Reform (progressive and liberal).[1] These branches have a wide variety of beliefs. That is why it is important to have a cleric of the same tradition as a patient.

Sacred writings are the Tanakh (the Hebrew Scripture as a whole, including the Torah—the first five books of the Bible); the Mishnah (regulations connected with Jewish life); and the Talmud (rabbinic teaching on the Tanakh and Mishnah).[2]

BELIEFS

Important Jewish themes are creation, revelation, and redemption. God's breath created the world from nothing.[3] The world was created good. Human inability to trust God resulted in sin and then death. Despite this, God desires human beings to be his co-creators. They do this by following God's commandments (*mitzvot*), which were given to Moses on Mt. Sinai, and walking in God's way (*halakhah*).[4]

Religious Jews pray three times each day (or more), observe the Sabbath (sundown on Friday until sundown on Saturday), and follow the kosher dietary laws.[5]

Basic Jewish beliefs are (1) God is transcendent but omnipresent (divine presence); (2) God is timeless and eternal; (3) God is omniscient and omnipotent; (4) Israel was elected by God as the chosen people; (5) the Torah is God's revelation; (6) failure to obey God is a sin; and (7) Jewish eschatology includes a Messiah who will come to usher in an era of peace, the rebuilding of Jerusalem, the resurrection of the dead, and the final judgment. The "messianic age" will follow a time of calamity that will lead to world peace and perfect societies. When the dead are resurrected, body and soul will be rejoined. If one's good actions outweigh one's evil deeds, a heavenly eternity awaits; if the evil outweighs the good, Gehenna, a place of torment, awaits.[6]

In terms of the Messiah, the Orthodox believe in a personal Messiah, while other branches believe in a collective messianic age in which human beings are enlightened. Similarly, in terms of resurrection, the Orthodox believe in a bodily resurrection and physical life after death with the coming of the Messiah; until that time, the righteous wait in "the world to come" while the evil go to Gehenna. The Conservative believe that there will be a physical raising of the dead when the Messiah comes. The Reconstructionists believe that there is no bodily resurrection, and that after death, the soul returns to the universe. Finally, the Reformed believe that there is no bodily resurrection or physical life after death, but that the soul, which is immortal, returns to God at death. Only the Reformed accept flowers at the funeral of one of their members.[7]

ILLNESS AND DEATH: IDEAL PRACTICES

An ill person should not be left alone but should be accompanied by family members. All Jews, however, are called to visit the ill, but a rabbi of the ill person's same tradition should be called. Death can never be hastened (i.e., no euthanasia), but extraordinary measures can be refused.[8] God is the Physician who created physicians, so physicians are to be respected.

Although Hasidic and Orthodox Jews do not permit autopsy or cremation, the other branches of Judaism vary in their approaches to these issues. Also, many Jews, regardless of branch, will permit organ donation if it will directly benefit another human being. It is believed that a "good" death is one in which the dying person has lived a long life, is surrounded by loved ones, or is at home. It is a blessing to die on the eve of the Sabbath or during the High Holy Days.[9] As a person is dying, he or she can confess his or her sins to God directly. At death, the dying or mourners pray the Shema ("Hear, O Israel, the Lord, our God is one!").[10]

At death, the entire body should be straightened out; bloodstained bed linens should be buried with the body.[11] The mouth and eyes are closed and the lower jaw is bound to the head.[12] Hasidic and Orthodox Jews insist that a member of their tradition prepare the body for burial. Preparation includes ritually washing the body, dressing it in white clothes or a shroud (a sign of humility). The body is never left alone until burial occurs. The body cannot be moved on a Sabbath. Some Jews place the body (covered with a sheet) on the floor with feet toward the door and a candle by the head. Orthodox Jews place the body in a pine box. Embalming is not permitted.[13]

The funeral is fifteen to sixty minutes in length and is within twenty-four hours of death (unless it is a Sabbath) at a synagogue or funeral home. At the service, a rabbi leads, a cantor sings, and a memorial *kaddish* (prayer of praise) is recited. Psalms, prayers, and eulogies are offered. Mourners make a small tear in their clothes or on a special ribbon (worn on their right lapel) as a sign of grief. The meaning is that just as the ribbon (or clothes) are torn, the deceased is torn away from his or her family. Only family and close friends go to the gravesite, where the mourners throw a spadeful of dirt into the grave as the casket is lowered into the ground.[14] Friends and neighbors sit *shiva* ("seven") with the family for seven days after the funeral, mourning with them at home and attending to their needs; this is not done on the Sabbath, which is meant to be a day of joy. Family members sit on floor or low stools, as a sign of humility.[15] They also cover mirrors, burn a special memorial candle, wear socks but no shoes, do not shave (men), and have a prayer service (*kaddish*) twice each day for ten to twenty minutes every morning and evening. The *yahrzeit* candle burns all seven days.[16]

Several anniversaries of the death are important in the Jewish tradition. For eleven months after the death of a parent or child, mourners attend daily morning and evening services at a synagogue or temple, where the mourners recite a special *kaddish*. At the one-year anniversary, there is a special service at the synagogue or temple. At the deceased's home, a *yahrzeit* candle burns twenty-four hours, and at the burial site, the tombstone is unveiled.[17]

MODIFICATIONS ON IDEAL JEWISH PRACTICES BASED ON WESTERN MEDICAL ROUTINES

Death can never be hastened (i.e., no euthanasia), but extraordinary measures can be refused. Although Hasidic and Orthodox Jews do not permit autopsy or cremation, the other branches of Judaism vary in their approaches to these issues. Also, many Jews, regardless of branch, now permit organ donation as a gift of life to another person.

ILLNESS AND DEATH IN CHILDREN

There are no specific prayers or practices for children that are different from those for adults. A viable infant is one who has lived for at least thirty days, and the mourning practices for such a child would be the same as for an adult. Infants who live less than thirty days or who are stillborn and fetuses (i.e., miscarriages) are not considered viable and would not be entitled to the same mourning periods as are adults, teens, children, and infants who have lived for at least thirty days. When infants live for less than thirty days or are stillborn or still fetuses, Jewish tradition holds that their soul was only temporarily on earth and returns to heaven from where we believe all souls emanate.[18]

Jewish children are traditionally buried in a separate section of a Jewish cemetery dedicated to children, although, in some cases, they can be buried with adults.

Prayers

The traditional Jewish prayer for the ill is the *Mishabairach*:

May the One who blessed our forefathers Abraham, Isaac, and Jacob, and our foremothers Sarah, Rebecca, Rachel, and Leah, bless and heal [NAME], the son/daughter of [NAMES]. May the Holy One, blessed be G-d, be merciful and strengthen and heal him/her. Grant him/her a complete and speedy recovery—healing of body and healing of soul, along with all the ill. And let us say Amen. ✌

Rebbe Nachman, an eighteenth-century mystic, offered this prayer for healing:

> God of wholeness, God of healing, Hear our words, Accept our prayers; Send a special blessing of healing to [NAME], son/daughter of [MOTHER'S NAME], among all those of Your children who are in need of Your healing blessing.[19] ✌

The Psalms are a wonderful treasury of prayers for those who are ill, dying, or in need. Especially helpful are Psalms 22, 23, 38, 41, 71 (for those of old age), and 88. Among these, Psalms 23, 41, and 71 convey hope, whereas Psalms 22, 38, and 88 describe feelings that the ill person may have.

The same prayers that are said for adults are said for children: for ill children, the Psalms (especially Psalm 23) and the *Mishabairach*; and for the dead, the *Kali Malai*.[20] At death, the dying or mourners pray the Shema ("Hear, O Israel, the Lord, our God is one!"). There should be no Christian blessings or anointing, and the name of Jesus should not be invoked.

The *Kali Malai* is said for one who has died:

⋮ O G-d, full of compassion, Who dwells on
⋮ high, grant perfect rest beneath the shadow
of thy divine presence in the exalted places
among the holy and pure, who shine like the
glow of the firmament for the soul of [NAME],
who went on to his/her eternal home. In the
merit that we remember them and recall all
their good deeds. May You, O G-d of mercy,
shelter him/her forever under the wings of Your
divine presence. May his/her soul be bound up
in the bond of life eternal, and grant that his/
her memories ever inspire us always to a noble
and consecrated living. Amen.[21] ❧

CONCLUDING
THOUGHTS

....

WHEN MY STUDENTS stumped me with questions
I could not answer, I embarked on a quest to learn
more about the beliefs of five major world religions
and how those beliefs informed the prayers and practices at the times of illness, death, and loss. I have been
rewarded in a number of ways. First of all, I learned a
great deal and now better understand why the various religions do what they do. Certain practices still
might seem foreign to me, but I can now appreci-
ate the practices' meanings and roles at the time of
illness, death, or loss for those who adhere to those
religious traditions. Second, I became more sensitive
to those who don't share my beliefs and am willing
to show them hospitality. After all, if this is the way

that they encounter God, who am I to complain or judge? Third, I have embraced my own faith tradition more deeply. By hearing about others' beliefs, prayers, and practices, I did not become confused. Instead, the quest prompted me to better understand the meaning of prayers and practices in my own tradition. In the end, I was graced in ways beyond my imagination when I started this endeavor.

Prejudice arises out of fear, and fear arises out of ignorance. When we don't know others or their beliefs or practices, we fear them because they are strange to us. Out of our fear, we often draw conclusions about them, conclusions that are frequently erroneous. These conclusions can lead to prejudice, which can affect the way we view the world and the many peoples in it. These prejudices can cause immeasurable harm, on both individual and global levels.

We who believe in God must acknowledge that we do not fully understand why God encounters people in so many different ways. But that is precisely what God does. Someone across the globe may love God as much or even more than I do, but express it very differently than I do. Someone in my own neighborhood may do good deeds or act charitably for reasons very different from the reasons that I do good deeds or act charitably. Such differences are the reality of our world. Rather than speculating about whose way is better—especially in times of illness, death, suffering, or loss—let us move forward, granting others the dignity that we would have them grant us.

NOTES

....

1. Buddhism

1. Christopher Partridge, ed., *Introduction to World Religions* (Minneapolis, MN: Fortress Press, 2005), 189.
2. Ibid., 195.
3. Kenneth Kramer, *The Sacred Art of Dying* (Mahwah, NJ: Paulist Press, 1988), 50.
4. Ibid., 64.
5. Partridge, *Introduction to World Religions*, 202.
6. Ibid.
7. Neville Kirkwood, *A Hospital Handbook on Multiculturalism and Religion* (Harrisburg, PA: Morehouse Publishing, 1993), 84.
8. Partridge, *Introduction to World Religions*, 199.
9. Kirkwood, *Hospital Handbook*, 84.
10. Partridge, *Introduction to World Religions*, 201.
11. Kirkwood, *Hospital Handbook*, 87.
12. Kramer, *Sacred Art of Dying*, 54.

13. Mary Toole, *Handbook for Chaplains* (Mahwah, NJ: Paulist Press, 2006), 3.

14. Kramer, *Sacred Art of Dying*, 54.

15. Kathleen Garces-Foley, ed., *Death and Religion in a Changing World* (Armonk, NY: M. E. Sharpe, 2006), 79, and Kramer, *Sacred Art of Dying*, 53.

16. Toole, *Handbook for Chaplains*, 3.

17. Kramer, *Sacred Art of Dying*, 76–78.

18. Ibid., 66.

19. Toole, *Handbook for Chaplains*, 3.

20. Garces-Foley, *Death and Religion*, 76.

21. Kramer, *Sacred Art of Dying*, 54.

22. Stuart Matlins, *The Perfect Stranger's Guide to Funerals and Grieving Practices* (Woodstock, VT: SkyLight Paths Publishing, 2000), 40–42.

23. Kirkwood, *Hospital Handbook*, 88–89.

24. Kramer, *Sacred Art of Dying*, 54.

25. Garces-Foley, *Death and Religion*, 74.

26. Ibid., 79.

27. Matlins, *The Perfect Stranger's Guide*, 44.

28. Thich Nhat Hanh, *Plum Village Chanting and Recitation Book* (Berkeley, CA: Parallax Press, 2000), 180–85. Reprinted with permission of Parallax Press, www.parallax.org.

29. Ibid., 180.

30. Ibid., 182.

31. Ibid., 183–84.

32. Ibid., 184–85.

33. Ibid., 185.

34. Ibid., 194–98.

2. Christianity

1. Kenneth Kramer, *The Sacred Art of Dying* (Mahwah, NJ: Paulist Press, 1988), 152.

2. Neville Kirkwood, *A Hospital Handbook on Multicultur-alism and Religion*, (Harrisburg, PA: Morehouse Publishing, 1993), 22.

3. Ibid., 24.

4. Ibid., 20.

5. Ibid., 23.

6. Mary Toole, *Handbook for Chaplains* (Mahwah, NJ: Paulist Press, 2006), 47.

7. Ibid.

8. The Episcopal Church, *The Book of Common Prayer* (New York: Seabury Press, 1979), 458.

9. Ibid., 458–59.

10. Ibid., 494.

11. Ibid.

12. *Occasional Services: A Companion to the Lutheran Book of Worship* (Minneapolis: Augsburg Publishing House, 1997), 92–93.

13. Ibid., 56.

14. *The United Methodist Book of Worship* (Nashville: Abingdon Press, 1992), 621. A Service of Healing I and A Service of Healing II ©1992 The United Methodist Publishing House. Used by Permission.

15. Ibid., 166. ©1992 The United Methodist Publishing House. Used by Permission.

16. Ibid, 167. ©1992 The United Methodist Publishing House. Used by Permission.

17. Ibid., 162. ©1992 The United Methodist Publishing House. Used by Permission.

18. *The Methodist Worship Book* (Peterborough, UK: Methodist Publishing House, 1999), 482.

19. Ibid., 486.

20. Peter Gregory, *Transfiguration Orthodox Prayer Book*, http://www.transchurch.org/sguide/prayerbook.asp (accessed August 3, 2007).

21. Ibid.

22. Ibid.

23. *Prayers and Meditations for the Sick and the Suffering* (Syosset, NY: Orthodox Church in America, 1983). Reprinted in *Prayers in Time of Sickness, Suffering, Dying and Death*, http://yya.oca.org/TheHub/Prayers/Prayer BookletSicknessDeath.pdf (accessed August 3, 2007).

24. Gregory, *Transfiguration Orthodox Prayer Book.*

25. *Orthodox Prayer Book* (Holy Protection Orthodox Monastery: New Veratic Publishing, 1990). Reprinted in *Prayers in Time of Sickness, Suffering, Dying and Death*, http://yya.oca.org/TheHub/Prayers/PrayerBookletSick nessDeath.pdf (accessed August 3, 2007).

26. There are numerous versions of the Trisagion prayers. This one is from www.orthodoxwiki.org/Trisagion (accessed 9/2/2007).

27. Theology and Worship Ministry Unit, *Presbyterian Book of Common Worship* (Louisville, KY: Westminster/John Knox Press, 1993), 988.

28. Ibid., 830.

29. Ibid., 989.

30. Ibid., 988.

31. Ibid., 1028.

32. International Commission on English in the Liturgy, *Pastoral Care of the Sick* (New York: Catholic Book Publishing Co., 1983), 43.

33. Ibid., 52–55.

34. International Commission on English in the Liturgy, *Order of Christian Funerals* (Chicago: Liturgy Training Publications, 1989), 141.

35. Ibid., 142.

3. Hinduism

1. Christopher Partridge, ed., *Introduction to World Religions* (Minneapolis, MN: Fortress Press, 2005), 137.

2. Ibid., 149.

3. Neville Kirkwood, *A Hospital Handbook on Multiculturalism and Religion* (Harrisburg, PA: Morehouse Publishing, 1993), 62–63.

4. Ibid., 64.

5. Partridge, *Introduction to World Religions*, 146–48.

6. Stuart Matlins, *The Perfect Stranger's Guide to Funerals and Grieving Practices* (Woodstock, VT: SkyLight Paths Publishing, 2000), 97.

7. Kramer, *Sacred Art of Dying*, 30.

8. Matlins, *The Perfect Stranger's Guide*, 30–31.

9. Kramer, *Sacred Art of Dying*, 36.

10. Ibid., 35.

11. Kirkwood, *Hospital Handbook*, 69.

12. Mary Toole, *Handbook for Chaplains* (Mahwah, NJ: Paulist Press, 2006), 16.

13. Kirkwood, *Hospital Handbook*, 69–70; Kathleen Garces-Foley, ed., *Death and Religion in a Changing World* (Armonk, NY: M. E. Sharpe, 2006), 30; and Kramer, *Sacred Art of Dying*, 39.

14. Garces-Foley, *Death and Religion*, 31.

15. Kramer, *Sacred Art of Dying*, 39.

16. Matlins, *The Perfect Stranger's Guide*, 98–99.

17. Kramer, *Sacred Art of Dying*, 39.

18. Garces-Foley, *Death and Religion*, 32.

19. Ibid., 33.

20. Kramer, *Sacred Art of Dying*, 39.

21. Garces-Foley, *Death and Religion*, 39.

22. Ibid., 39–40.

23. Ibid., 39.

24. Kumar Bhattacharya, e-mail message, March 18, 2007.
25. Juan Mascaro, trans., *The Bhagavad Gita* (New York: Penguin Books, 1962).

4. Islam

1. Christopher Partridge, ed., *Introduction to World Religions* (Minneapolis, MN: Fortress Press, 2005), 358.
2. Ibid., 363.
3. Neville Kirkwood, *A Hospital Handbook on Multiculturalism and Religion* (Harrisburg, PA: Morehouse Publishing, 1993), 37.
4. Partridge, *Introduction to World Religions*, 372–75.
5. Ibid., 376–81.
6. Kenneth Kramer, *The Sacred Art of Dying* (Mahwah, NJ: Paulist Press, 1988), 162.
7. Kramer, *Sacred Art of Dying*, 160–63; Kathleen Garces-Foley, ed., *Death and Religion in a Changing World*. (Armonk, NY: M. E. Sharpe, 2006), 154–58; and Partridge, *Introduction to World Religions*, 375.
8. Kramer, *Sacred Art of Dying*, 164.
9. Ibid., 163.
10. Ibid.
11. Kirkwood, *Hospital Handbook*, 39–40.
12. Ibid., 43.
13. Mary Toole, *Handbook for Chaplains* (Mahwah, NJ: Paulist Press, 2006), 26.
14. Kirkwood, *Hospital Handbook*, 44.
15. Kramer, *Sacred Art of Dying*, 166.
16. Kirkwood, *Hospital Handbook*, 41.
17. Ibid., 45.
18. Dr. Nour Akhras, e-mail message to author, December 27, 2006.
19. Garces-Foley, *Death and Religion*, 162.
20. Stuart Matlins, *The Perfect Stranger's Guide to Funerals*

    and Grieving Practices (Woodstock, VT: SkyLight Paths Publishing, 2000), 114–15.

21. Garces-Foley, *Death and Religion*, 162–63.
22. Ibid., 163.
23. Kirkwood, *Pastoral Care to Muslims*, 131–32.
24. Ibid., 132.
25. Ibid., 132–33.
26. Ibid., 133.
27. Ibid., 133.
28. Akhras, e-mail message to author, December 27, 2006.
29. Ibid.

5. Judaism

1. Christopher Partridge, ed., *Introduction to World Religions* (Minneapolis, MN: Fortress Press, 2005), 273–76.
2. Ibid., 282–86.
3. Kenneth Kramer, *The Sacred Art of Dying* (Mahwah, NJ: Paulist Press, 1988), 127.
4. Partridge, *Introduction to World Religions*, 294–95.
5. Ibid., 290–94.
6. Ibid., 286–89.
7. Stuart Matlins, *The Perfect Stranger's Guide to Funerals and Grieving Practices* (Woodstock, VT: SkyLight Paths Publishing, 2000), 126.
8. Neville Kirkwood, *A Hospital Handbook on Multiculturalism and Religion* (Harrisburg, PA: Morehouse Publishing, 1993), 54.
9. Kathleen Garces-Foley, ed., *Death and Religion in a Changing World* (Armonk, NY: M. E. Sharpe, 2006), 53.
10. Kramer, *Sacred Art of Dying*, 135.
11. Mary Toole, *Handbook for Chaplains* (Mahwah, NJ: Paulist Press, 2006), 36.
12. Kramer, *Sacred Art of Dying*, 135.

13. Kirkwood, *Hospital Handbook*, 56, and Garces-Foley, *Death and Religion*, 56.
14. Matlins, *The Perfect Stranger's Guide*, 126–29; Kramer, *Sacred Art of Dying*, 135; Partridge, *Introduction to World Religions*, 293–94.
15. Kramer, *Sacred Art of Dying*, 135.
16. Matlins, *The Perfect Stranger's Guide*, 129; Kramer, *Sacred Art of Dying*, 135; Garces-Foley, *Death and Religion*, 60–61.
17. Matlins, *The Perfect Stranger's Guide*, 130.
18. Rabbi Schur, telephone conversation, November 17, 2006.
19. Rebbe Nachman of Breslov, "Prayer for Healing," www.bikurcholimcc.org/visiting4.html (accessed March 22, 2008).
20. Rabbi Schur, e-mail message to author, March 24, 2008.
21. Ibid.

BIBLIOGRAPHY

Garces-Foley, Kathleen, ed. *Death and Religion in a Changing World*. Armonk, NY: M. E. Sharpe, 2006.

Kirkwood, Neville. *A Hospital Handbook on Multiculturalism and Religion*. Harrisburg, PA: Morehouse Publishing, 1993.

———. *Pastoral Care to Muslims*. New York: Haworth Press, 2002.

Kramer, Kenneth. *The Sacred Art of Dying*. Mahwah, NJ: Paulist Press, 1988.

Mascaro, Juan, trans. *The Bhagavad Gita*. New York: Penguin Books, 1962.

Matlins, Stuart, ed. *The Perfect Stranger's Guide to Funerals and Grieving Practices*. Woodstock, VT: SkyLight Paths Publishing, 2000.

Nhat Hanh, Thich. *Plum Village Chanting and Recitation Book*. Berkeley, CA: Parallax Press, 2000.

Partridge, Christopher, ed. *Introduction to World Religions.* Minneapolis, MN: Fortress Press, 2005.

Toole, Mary. *Handbook for Chaplains.* Mahwah, NJ: Paulist Press, 2006.